Top 10 Tips

for a Healthy Mind, Body and Soul

How to Practice Self-Care and Feel More Connected to Yourself and the World Around You

To Mom,

who made it all possible.

Table of Contents

Introduction

We've all heard the cliché "health is wealth", and although it's true, I'd like to add another layer of truth to that statement. Not only is our health our wealth, it is our *life*.

No matter how beautiful, intelligent, wealthy, or sexy you may be, if you do not prioritize your health, you will struggle in life. That's why this book focuses on the top ten simple self-care practices that will improve your health and, therefore, change your life.

Of course, there are more than ten self-care practices that you can engage in, but the tips you will encounter in this book are the most practical and simple tips that will add incredible value to your daily life.

Without spending too much time in the introductory section, let's begin our journey to health and complete wellness with the first practice. Can you guess what the first practice is? Take a deep breath, relax, and meditate!

Chapter One
Meditate Regularly

When some people think of meditation, images of a bald-headed monk wrapped in orange robes and sitting cross-legged on a mountaintop may come to mind. However, meditation doesn't need to be such a mystical thing. It can actually be a very simple, practical strategy to achieve greater calmness and focus in life.

There is a deep connection between the mind, body, and soul. That's why stress and depression make it difficult to stay well. So to take care of the body, you must first take care of the mind, and meditation is a great way to do so.

However, the key here isn't just to *meditate,* it is to meditate *regularly*. Some people meditate once in a while and wonder why they are still not at complete and utter peace with themselves. Well, all good things take time, and the real benefits won't be seen until a regular practice is established.

In the beginning, try to meditate for at least 5 minutes around the same time each day. Choosing a similar time daily will make it easier for your meditation practice to become habit. The more often you sit in stillness, the easier it will be for you to set aside this time for yourself. As it becomes more comfortable, you can slowly increase the time you meditate to 10, 15, or 20 minutes at a time.

There are many different kinds of meditation, each having its own set of benefits. For most people, mindfulness meditation is an excellent place to start[1]. Simply find a quiet place, sit comfortably, set a timer, and turn your attention to *one* object of focus - the sounds around you, your breath, or the thoughts in your mind. It is natural for the mind to wander, and when it does, gently return your attention to the object of focus.

One misconception about meditation is that we should try to stop the thoughts in our mind, and that if we can't stop our thoughts that we are somehow "bad" at meditating. This is simply not true. The goal should just be to focus on one thing. When the mind wanders, as it naturally does, we return to our object of focus. Every time we do this, it acts as a sort of "push-up" for the mind, and meditation becomes easier over time.

Have you been feeling overwhelmed lately? Are you stressed out? Do you feel like there are so many things you want to do and yet you feel exhausted and constrained? Is your mind restless, even when it's time to sleep? What you need is to establish a consistent meditation practice that will set your mind at ease.

Meditation isn't the first tip in the book by coincidence. It is the first tip because life is lived from the inside out and the state of your mind largely determines the state of your body and overall health.

Take a proactive first step by meditating today. Pick a quiet time in your day and separate yourself from others as you work to de-clutter your mind and find peace in stillness.

Chapter Two

Get Regular, Quality Sleep

The importance of regular, quality sleep cannot be overstated. If you are having issues with your health or struggling with any other physical, mental, or emotional challenge, make sure your sleep is a priority.

Think of your body as a machine; it works every second as you try to achieve your tasks and goals throughout the day, week, month or even year. Even machines need to have moments of rest or break-time; else they will break down. The same goes for your body.

We live in a society that values hard work and success over nearly everything else, and we are often praised for our accomplishments no matter what we had to do to get there. Contrary to popular opinion, rest isn't a luxury;

nor should it be a bragging right to sleep less than, say, 6 hours per night. Your body needs about eight hours of sleep nightly, anything less than that will affect you negatively.

Improved sleep quality has been tied to many health benefits including improved cognition, faster reflexes, increased productivity, and improved mental health[2]. It even offers a protective benefit to help you maintain a normal body weight. Knowing these benefits, you should be excited about rest, and that excitement should drive you to have a sleep routine that you stick to regardless of what happens during the day. Don't sacrifice quality sleep for anything.

A great way to improve sleep consistency and quality is to establish a night-time ritual. Night-time rituals can differ from person to person, and often there's a period of time involved to find out what works best for you. Many night-time rituals involve staying away from screens for an hour before bed, writing in a gratitude journal, doing your skincare routine, doing yoga or stretching, or drinking a cup of herbal tea before bed.

Many people, as a part of their night-time routine, also engage in jade rolling. A jade roller is a massage tool for the face with roots in ancient Chinese tradition and scientifically proven benefits when used regularly. Among these benefits are a brighter complexion, reduction of under-eye bags and dark circles, and a reduction in the appearance of fine lines and wrinkles[3]. It is an excellent addition to any night-time routine and functions not only as a beauty tool but also as a stress reliever and relaxation tool.

In the previous chapter, we focused on meditation but with emphasis on *regular* meditation. In this chapter, we focus on sleep but with an emphasis on *quality*. Aim to sleep well enough (and long enough) for your brain and body to be rejuvenated for the long haul.

When we wake up from sleep in the morning, after our various morning rituals, we often race to the kitchen for breakfast, and maybe coffee, to get our day started. In the next chapter, we'll look at the kinds of food to include (and exclude!) from your plate to start your day off on the right foot.

Chapter Three

Eat More Plant-Based Foods

In the previous section, we talked about how the human body is like a machine. As with all machines, there are certain things required to function effectively. For human beings, among the most important things we require to operate at our best are healthy, whole foods.

Food is fuel for the body; it is the single most important ingredient needed to refuel our bodies other than water and maybe the occasional nutritional supplement. Because food is our fuel, we can't eat just anything. The foods we choose to consume have a tremendous impact on our mood, our weight, our heart health, and our susceptibility to certain diseases[4].

Our world has evolved a lot, and now more than ever, people are seeking the "fast lane" of pre-packaged, over-processed fast food and drinks. Seemingly a great solution for the busy and hardworking person, these fast foods are actually more detrimental to our health than anything, and do not add any value whatsoever.

It's time we look to the past to try and see a better way forward. Although *most* things have improved since the days before mass food industrialization, we still have a lot to learn from past generations and how they used to cook and eat.

Before modern-day food industrialization, pre-packaging and calorie-counting, people only had simple rules to follow to try to maintain a healthy diet. One of the best and simplest rules is to "eat a rainbow" of nutrients and colors. Your plate should always be filled with a variety of colorful and flavorful foods that add minerals and nutrients to your body.

Another great tip is to eat local. Eating local is important for a number of reasons. First, your food won't have to travel as far before it reaches your plate, so there will be less preservatives and chemicals used in order to keep it fresh. Second, fresher food tastes better. You can definitely taste the difference between a freshly picked apple and an apple picked two weeks ago, wrapped in plastic, and transported from miles away. Third, eating locally allows you to reduce your carbon footprint and your impact on the environment.

We should all eat more fruits, vegetables, and foods that are free from chemicals and other unhealthy additives. In other words, *whole* foods. Instead of taking a strict and rigorous approach to the foods you eat, try to follow a few simple rules that are easy to stick with. For example:

1. Drink a glass of water half an hour before each meal
2. Eat lots of fiber
3. Enjoy your food slowly and mindfully
4. Eat locally
5. Eat a rainbow of nutrients and colors

Choosing one or two simple rules to follow helps guarantee that you will stick with your new diet - because as with anything pertaining to health, consistency is key.

As always, consult your doctor before making changes to your diet, but as a general rule, our diets should be free from unnatural additives like pesticides, hormones, and food dyes that are not healthy. Even when you're out with friends or family, be mindful to feed your body with the right kind of fuel.

Chapter Four

Read and Learn Often

Reading stimulates the mind - but more than that, it helps you stay vitalized with knowledge. Your brain needs to be cared for and nurtured in order for you to stay level-headed and sharp. Therefore, the best way to "feed" your brain is to read regularly and always continue the pursuit of knowledge.

We can never read too many books. Some people even believe that the answers to the problems currently facing the world lie in books. When we open a book, we embark on a journey into its pages and give our minds a short break from the stressors of our daily lives. We close the book feeling inspired, refreshed and rejuvenated.

Studies have shown that reading reduces stress levels by about 68%[5]; it preserves brain health and lowers the risk of degenerative diseases like Alzheimer's and Dementia. When you read often, you will also be able to alleviate feelings of anxiety and depression while filling your brain with a variety of interesting subject matter.

So what do we recommend? Reading for 30 minutes daily is a good start for anyone, and you can build on that by slowly increasing the amount of time you read each day. Technology has made learning easier now with eBooks that can be bought or downloaded to your mobile device as you read on the go.

As you read, you will most likely come to discover a topic that you're extremely passionate about. This can be anything from fashion design to fitness. But discovering your passion isn't enough, you also need to fuel your passion, and we'll discuss that in the next chapter.

Chapter Five

Fuel Your Passion

We all know what passionate people look like. They look just like you and I but with a bit more "oomph" behind everything they say and do. These people approach every day as an exciting, new opportunity and inspire that feeling in those around them. Most of us deeply admire this quality in others and hope to manifest more of it in ourselves. Well, there are very simple ways to do this, but first we need to understand what passion is.

What is passion? Passion is what sets your soul on fire. It could be anything; all that matters is that it feels right for you. Some of us may know exactly what our passion is, others may need to do a bit more self-discovery before we find our "thing".

A great way to re-discover your passion is to look back at your childhood. Try to remember what you did as a kid that you could do for hours without feeling bored. Did you build things? Write imaginative, short stories? How about take things apart just to put them back together again?

When you find an activity you used to enjoy as a child, try re-integrating it into your life now. The process of discovering your passion might take a while and will probably involve some trial and error, but don't give up! Keep on searching until you find something that makes you feel like a kid again.

Here are a few practical tips to make sure you're living a life fueled by passion.

1. **Seek satisfaction**

Too many people do certain things just because they have to. Although often necessary, this can also be frustrating. Whenever possible, focus on seeking comfort, passion, and joy. Only this can lead to a satisfied life.

2. Always do what you love

At least once a day, do something that you love. It can be blasting your favorite song in your car on the way to work, petting a fluffy dog that you pass by on the street, or watching one episode of your favorite show on TV. These things may not seem vital and you might go many days without doing anything to ignite your inner spark; but keep in mind that doing what you love is a form of self-care for the soul.

3. Be innovative with what you love

The world is continually evolving so if you want to stay at the peak of your passion you need to be creative with it.

Change with the times and seek different ways of doing what you love. If you are passionate about making people laugh, for example, you could create a YouTube channel or a website to share your humor with the world. Take advantage of modern trends and technologies to help share your gift with others.

A passion-filled life will always be an exciting one, it will lead you to places you never thought you would go, but most importantly, it will help you feel grateful for life.

Chapter Six

Practice Gratitude

Practicing gratitude changes our lives in a number of incredible ways. I could dedicate an entire book just to the subject of gratitude and there would still be more to say. Simply put, practicing gratitude is crucial to having a happy and healthy mind. When we practice gratitude regularly, we can actually rewire our brains to see the world in a more positive light.

The benefits of practicing gratitude are numerous, so let's get right to a few of them.

Why should you practice gratitude for self-care?

1. It improves physical health

Scientific evidence shows that increased happiness is correlated with a stronger immune system, improved physical health, and even an increased tolerance for stress and other negative emotions[6].

2. Improves self-esteem

Gratitude for what you have and envy of others cannot coexist; therefore, the best way to banish jealous, negative feelings is to practice gratitude. When we feel grateful for what we have, we stop comparing ourselves to others.

3. You will sleep better

When we worry constantly, these same feelings of dread can follow us into bed at night. We then toss and turn with worry and stress and end up having a terrible night's sleep. Being grateful for even the smallest things throughout your day can help you get better quality sleep at night.

4.   It takes the pressure off

Many of us voluntarily torture ourselves with the things we *should* do, or *could* have. When we practice gratitude, we focus less on what we could have and more on what we have already. This frees us from pressure to become something else by forcing us to appreciate where we are at the moment.

Here's some quick tips to help you get started with gratitude:

1. When you wake every morning, say thank you for a new day and when you're ready to sleep at night, say thank you for a beautiful day regardless of how your day unfolded.

2. Get a gratitude journal. There is no right or wrong way to keep a gratitude journal, but one of the most effective ways is to write one thing you're grateful for and then five reasons why you're grateful for it.

You'll notice an almost immediate improvement to your mood after you write in your gratitude journal. However, after some time it's likely your mood will return back to its "set point". In order to maintain the amazing mood-improvement effect of gratitude, a regular practice must be established. The more consistently you practice gratitude, the more often you'll find yourself in a state of contentment versus dissatisfaction. Studies have shown that gratitude is a skill we all can cultivate[7], so try to commit the practice to habit as soon as possible.

Gratitude opens the door for unlimited blessings, peace, and contentment in your life which makes it easier for you to enjoy other things you love. What are you grateful for today?

Chapter Seven

Find an Exercise You Enjoy

We all know that exercise is good for the body. Yet, despite this knowledge, most people still don't have a regular exercise routine in place. Why is that? Well, it's probably not that people don't *believe* in the benefits of exercise - it's that they haven't found an exercise routine they enjoy yet!

For some, the thought of going to the gym regularly is the stuff of nightmares. For others, the thought of a group fitness or yoga class brings on similar feelings of dread. If you don't *enjoy* the exercise you do, very likely, you simply won't do it.

You may be confused by the sheer number of different exercise options available. To simplify this often complicated and intimidating subject, the word "enjoy" was added to this chapter.

The overall goal of exercise is simple - get up, get moving, and increase your heart rate to make your body healthier and stronger. Therefore, there is no single "perfect" exercise for anyone and there are often numerous different kinds of exercise we can do to reach our fitness goals. Remember to always contact your doctor before making big changes to your exercise routine, but don't be afraid to try something new.

Exercise is inherently healthy for the body, but why not add fun and enjoyment to the mix? To do this, think back to the chapter about reigniting your passion and feeling like a kid again. Remember some of the things you used to do for fun back in the day. Then, try integrating some of these things into your exercise routine. This can be dance, a particular kind of music, spending time in nature, a need for speed (hello, runners and cyclists!), or being with friends. Even hula hoop and jump-rope are great exercises. Whatever it is, add elements of it into your fitness routine and you'll be significantly more likely to stick to it.

Exercise can be an outlet for negative emotions like anger and frustration. It's also an excellent time to "check in" with yourself and evaluate your overall internal well-being. When we exercise, we take our minds off of our problems and can reemerge after our workout more energized to tackle them. In these ways, exercise is self-care for the entire body - inside and out.

If you have struggled with exercise in the past, the best thing to do is keep it simple. You can start with a simple routine such as walking around the neighborhood. Your steps can become jogs overtime and then long hikes. You can also start with short at-home workouts and gradually increase the duration as your body gets stronger.

Self-care is all about taking preventative steps to care for our bodies and improve ourselves daily; that's why exercise is at the foundation of any good self-care routine.

Chapter Eight

Spend Time outside every day

When did you last make it to the beach? The park? Or even take a walk around your neighborhood? Not all of us are lucky enough to live minutes away from a white sand beach or a majestic mountain range, but even a quick stroll around the block can improve your mood[8].

For those of us who come from cooler climates, going outside is something we simply tolerate for many months of the year, if not avoid entirely. But spending time outside gives us access to mother nature and all her wonderful gifts - fresh air, warm sun, sandy beaches, and beautiful mountains and forests, helping us feel a little more at peace.

These quiet moments in nature are a great time for a little self-care. People who spend large amounts of time outside can attest to the fact that being outdoors is almost always relaxing and restorative, and helps you maintain a calmer approach towards life.

Humans are inextricably tied to nature and yet most of us spend the vast majority of our time indoors. Many of us have hectic schedules, and our daily dealings with work and others can be stressful, so it's important to be intentional about spending time outside. Breathe in the fresh air, admire the trees, feel the sun on your skin, and relax from the stressors of modern life.

Time spent outside is excellent for introspection and reflection; and reflection is an opportunity for you to make positive changes in the areas of your life that need adjusting. If you need an outlet to document all of your important thoughts and realizations, try starting with a daily journal.

Chapter Nine

Keep a Journal

Keeping a journal is always a good idea; it helps you keep tabs on yourself and everything that happens around you. The reason a lot of people feel disappointed in life is because they lack clarity - a critical component of happiness. A journal allows you to clear the clutter in your mind as well as keep track of your accomplishments and setbacks, and put the events of your life (good and bad) into perspective.

When we lack clarity, we often feel aimless and unaccomplished, and this can be a difficult feeling to deal with. Writing often in your journal helps you have a better connection with your values, emotions, and goals; and if you ever lose sight of the bigger picture you'll be able to get back on track to personal happiness with ease.

With a journal, you'll experience improved mental clarity that sharpens problem solving abilities and overall focus. Increased understanding of yourself and the ability to track your personal development are some of the additional benefits that come with keeping a journal[9].

We should all be thankful for technology as it has paved the way for things like journaling to be done more comfortably. Instead of having to keep a journal on you at all times, you can simply jot down journal entries into your phone as soon as inspiration strikes.

However, if you don't want to use a digital journal, you can always stick to a traditional journal; whichever works best for you. Refer back to it regularly in order to assess progress in key areas of your life.

All of the tips you have encountered thus far should be done regularly for maximum effect; journaling is no exception. If you run out of inspiration to write in your journal, go online and search "Journal prompts for [month]" and you'll find numerous prompts to help get the gears turning.

The journey toward self-care is worthwhile, but it won't always be easy. We may have setbacks, hurdles, and distractions along the way. Keep reading for the #10 tip about how to eliminate the biggest hurdle on your self-care journey.

Chapter Ten

Eliminate Distractions

Distraction comes in various forms; sometimes it comes from within you and other times it comes from others. Distractions are like blockages you experience when you're working on a great project; they crop up from within and around you, make you lose focus, and sometimes, without even realizing it, we give in to them.

The first step for anyone is to identify what your primary distractions are before working towards eliminating them. What may be a distraction for you may not be for someone else and vice versa, so an honest evaluation of ourselves is a crucial part of this first step.

Anything that makes it difficult for you to finish projects on time or accomplish your goals is a distraction. People, activities, places, and habits that deter your progress must go. Sometimes, these distractions are obvious. Loud music, a chatty coworker, or a phone that doesn't seem to stop buzzing are all examples of obvious distractions.

Other distractions, although less obvious, can have an equally detrimental effect on our productivity. Studies have shown that spending time with negative people can derail us from our goals and increase the likelihood that we will actually pick up new bad habits instead[10].

Follow these simple steps to ensure that your life is free from distraction:

1. **Put your phone on silent when it's time to work**. You may worry that you'll miss an important email or phone call if you put your phone on silent - but that likely won't happen.

Silence all notifications while you work so you can focus completely on the task at hand.

2. **Create blocks of time dedicated to certain activities, including break times as well.** Parkinson's law states that "work expands so as to fill the time available for its completion". This law, originally coined by C. Northcote Parkinson, has tremendous implications for productivity studies, and means that it's often better to set shorter windows of time to finish tasks rather than longer ones. Don't forget to block out break times as well.

3. **Prioritize what's on your to-do list and knock it out in order of importance.** Most people tend to "put off" doing the most dreaded activities until the very last minute. In order to maximize your productivity, knock out the most dreaded tasks *first*.

4. Eliminate or minimize negative people in your life. This one goes back to our previous point about how negative people can impact our ability to accomplish our goals. We've all heard the adage that we are the average of the five people we spend the most time with; so make sure you're selective about who's in your top 5.

Let's go back to the drawing board. Look at everything you've been trying to do recently, everything you have dedicated time and energy to. What seems to be holding you back?

Maybe you're spending too much time online; perhaps you are procrastinating or surrounding yourself with the wrong crowd. Be honest with yourself about what's holding you back, and work hard to make the necessary changes. With distractions out of the way, there will be little holding you back from accomplishing everything you want in life.

Chapter Eleven

Create a Morning and Evening Self-Care Routine

Would it really be a "top ten" list without a number 11 bonus tip? Keep reading the last tip (I promise this is the last one!) to see how morning and evening self-care routines can impact your life.

Some of the happiest and most successful people in the world have morning and evening routines that they stick to religiously, rain or shine[11]. Barack Obama has said that he starts every day with either a cardio or weight routine, then has breakfast with his daughters. Anna Wintour, editor-in-chief at Vogue, starts her day off with an hour of tennis at the Midtown Tennis Club in New York.

No two morning or evening routines are alike, nor should they be. Yours should reflect the goals and challenges unique to you and should change as your life changes.

Among the other morning activities of highly successful people are waking up early, eating a healthy breakfast, walking the dog, or sitting quietly in meditation. Although the specific activities may vary, the idea behind all morning routines is the same. The goal is to take a little time to take care of you, and set the tone for a happy and productive day.

You will find some self-care tips for the morning and evening below:

Mornings

- Wake up early every morning, use an alarm clock if you tend to oversleep.

- Drink lots of water before eating to rehydrate your body after a long night's rest.

- Take some time for exercise or meditation (yoga is an excellent way to gently wake the body).

- Write in your gratitude journal to start out with a positive mindset and encourage grateful thoughts throughout your day.

- Don't forget to have breakfast (this is the most important meal of the day).

Evenings

- Get back home and have a healthy dinner - enjoy your meal with family or friends if at all possible.

- Reflect on your day by deciding what to avoid the following day and what to encourage.

- If you have kids, put them to bed early enough that you have time to relax and get quality sleep.

- Open the curtains before going to sleep, so you can rise naturally with the sun.

- Engage in some rejuvenating activities such as sipping herbal tea, taking a warm bath, or jade rolling with your new jade roller.

As mentioned before, jade rolling is one of the best activities to relax as well as rejuvenate the body. It can be used in the morning to "wake up" the skin, or in the evening to relax tension away.

Try to implement these practices as soon as possible so you can commit this routine to habit right away. If you need a little push to help you take the right steps on your self-care journey, all the motivation you need is in the next chapter.

Conclusion

Start Today!

At this point I'd like to say congratulations for making it to the end of this book! By this point, you've learned a lot about self care. Some of this information may have been new; the rest may have been the reminder and the motivation you needed to make positive changes in your life. With your brain now buzzing about how to practice gratitude, reduce distractions, and make healthier choices, there is no better time to act than *now*.

Some people say that "knowledge is power", but I disagree. All this knowledge without practical application won't help you one bit. Until you apply this knowledge to your life, you have the equivalent of a collection of expensive luxury cars that you never drive - silly and foolish.

Too many people wait for the perfect time to act. They want the stars to align before taking that first step. Right now is the best time to do what needs to be done.

Don't wait for a perfect sunny day to head out for exercise, don't allow distractions to get the best of you before eliminating them and don't wait until adverse effects start to surface before you take steps for self-care.

Let's make a pact here with this chapter; that you will not delay the process and you will not make excuses. You will do the most with the time you've been given. You will exercise, do your morning and evening routines, sleep properly, eat well, and meditate while making positive adjustments to your life.

Remember this lesson as we bring the journey to a close; at the end of the day, it is *your* job to be kind to yourself and treat yourself right. Be your own best friend, adviser, and therapist who will care for yourself before caring for others.

Everything you need to take proper care of yourself has been given to you. It is time to act - your time is now.

Best Wishes,

Morgan Lilly

References

1 Mineo, Liz. "Less Stress, Clearer Thoughts with Mindfulness Meditation." *The Harvard Gazette*, Harvard University, 17 Apr. 2018

2 Twery, Michael, Ph.D. "Get Enough Sleep." *Healthfinder.gov*, U.S. Department of Health and Human Services, 18 July 2018

3 Norton, Allison. "Beauty Note: What Is a Jade Roller and Should I Be Using One?" *Lauren Conrad*, 25 May 2018

4 Simpkin, May. "The Actual Relationship between Nutrition and Health." *May Simpkin*, 12 Nov. 2017

5 Bestler, Bob. "Relax, Read a Book (or a Newspaper Column). Here's How It Could Help You Live Longer." *Myrtlebeachonline*, Myrtle Beach Sun News, 10 Aug. 2018

6 Newman, Kira. "Six Ways Happiness Is Good for Your Health." *Greater Good*, University of California, Berkeley, 28 July 2015

7 Scott, S.J. "How to Be Happy." *Happier Human*, 19 Feb. 2019

8 Martinez, Eliza. "Drop Everything and Take a Walk around the Block: How Walking Affects Your Mood ..." *Allwomenstalk*, 11 Apr. 2015

9 Nguyen, Thai. "10 Surprising Benefits Of Keeping A Journal." *HuffPost*, HuffPost, 7 Dec. 2017

[10] Stillman, Jessica. "Chronic Negativity Can Literally Kill You, Science Shows." *Inc.com*, Inc., 13 Oct. 2016

[11] Cantero-Gomez, Paloma. "Get The Seven Early Morning Routines Used By Highly Successful People." *Forbes*, Forbes Magazine, 18 Oct. 2018

.

Image Credits

*Front cover image by © Aphiraa Gowry,
www.aphiraa.com.*

*Back cover image by © Damischa Wilson at Roc City Art
Complex - Beloit, Wisconsin.*

www.ingramcontent.com/pod-product-compliance
Lightning Source LLC
Chambersburg PA
CBHW021039180526
45163CB00005B/2194